Evincepub Publishing

Nehru Nagar, Bilaspur, Chhattisgarh 495001
First Published by Evincepub Publishing 2021
Copyright © Authors 2021
All Rights Reserved.
ISBN: 978-93-5446-317-4

SANKALP

Mneumonics in ENT, opthal & PSM

Dr. Chandrashekhar Singh
Dr. Krishan Rajbhar

ACKNOWLEDGEMENT

I would like to convey my gratitude to following persons:

My parents – Mr. Jay kumar singh, Mrs. Sushila devi

My friends: I express my gratitude to Dr. pooja Gandhi (M.S. OBG, GMC Gwalior) and Dr. Karuna Tiwari (MD Anastheia MGM Medical college Indore) for moral support and and encouragement which helped me a lot in preparing this book,

I am highly grateful to Dr Pulkit Chaturvedi (MD Dermatology SMS Jaipur), Dr Rohit Bhurre (M.S. Ortho,GMC Nagpur), Dr Kreetika saini (MD dermatology BJMC Ahmedabad) Dr Anshul Agrawal (M.S. Surgery, MGM Indore), Dr Jushya Bhatia (MD Dermatology SAIMS Indore) Dr Pradeep Pathak (MS Ortho, PGI Rohtak), Dr Lokendra Thakur (MD Medicne SION Mumbai), Dr Dependra (MD Radioloy MGM Indore) Dr Khushboo gyanchandani (MD medicine Safdarjung Hospital), Dr Pankaj (MD Radiology MGM Indore), Dr Arpit Agrawal (MD Anasthesia MGM indore), Dr Ajay Dhanopeya (MS Ortho)

Thanks,
Dr Chandrashekhar Singh
MBBS, MS (Gen Surg),
UPSC IAS (Pre cleared)

ACKNOWLEDGEMENT

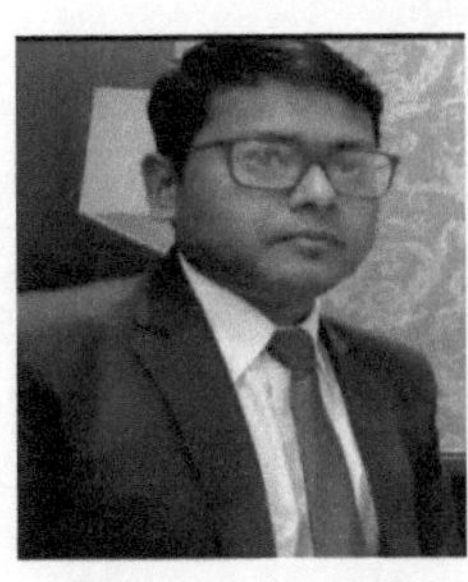

"My goal is not to be better than anyone else, but to be better than I used to be"
-Dr. Wayne W. Dyer

This is my 10th book for MBBS students, with an experience of authoring 45 books till now, I'm closer to my dream of 100 by 35, with each book I have tried to reform the content by manifolds and develop it further. This work having mnemonics of ENT, ophthalmology & community medicine which are third professional part 1 subjects & I find difficult to memorize lots of things during my days at VMMC!

This book has been the brainchild of my senior Dr. Chandrasekhar sir (I was his intern few years ago & I can vouch as he is one of the best seniors I have ever had), co-authoring a volume with him is a great privilege for me.

I am thankful to my entire family, Dr Poonam K Gedam, siblings - Dr. Sushil Rajbhar for their immense support in the times of need

My friends Dr. Sandeep (MD anesthesia), Dr. shivani (MS ENT), Dr. Paramita (MD OBG) are gem for me.

People at my department, Safdarjung hospital must be acknowledged to provide me sufficient clinical material for developing my clinical acumen

I must thank my family at Indian medical Association for supporting me Dr. Jayalal sir, Dr Karan juneja, Dr. Rahul anand & others.

Publishing team at Evince pub must be mentioned

Thanks, Dr Krishan Rajbhar
Resident ENT surgeon, Safdarjung hospital
Co- convenor, Indian medical
Association (JDN - NCR), Prolific author
to 45 medical books

PREFACE

I am most pleased to share with you my "this creativity", as you all know and you would have been realized till now the vast syllabus of MBBS. Syllabus is not only vast in size but it becomes very difficult to memorize the list of causes, symptom, signs, diseases etc, to overcome with this problem. I came with idea of creating mnemonics. I thought, this may be premature idea but after seeing the Pre-PG (now NEET PG) questions and answers, I felt, now its mandatory for me to make mnemonics. Because it was very difficult to memorize all pre-pg stuffs, so I created the mnemonics and I also believe that 'knowledge increases when we share it', I shared these mnemonics with my batch mates and seniors. They appreciated it very much so I come with this pocket book **SANKALP**" for PSM, OPHTHAL AND ENT (not published that time). And response was surprising!! Everyone was in need of tools like this. It helped me very much and I hope it would have helped all the readers .AND I hope it will help you too. Some people say one will need mnemonics to remember mnemonics but believe me you will need very less time to revise many topics and it will help to solve MCQs like anything and if you face any difficulty in memorizing any list, do not hesitate to share(cssingh1990@gmail.com) the list with me, I will make the best mnemonic for you.

Thank you, happy memorizing.

HEARING LOSS

SENSORINEURAL HEARING LOSS

CONGENITAL CAUSES OF SNHL

 **CoCHLeAR Nerve TRAUMA**

Co – Cockayne's syndrome*
C – Crouzon's D/S*
H – Hurlers syndrome
Le – Leopard Syndrome
A – Alport syndrome
R – Refsum syndrome
Nerve – Nail-patella   syndrome*
T – Treacher collin syndrome*
R – Renal tubular acidosis type-1*
A – Alstromsyndrome*
U – Usher syndrome
M – Michel's aplasia*
A – Albinism

 * - have been asked in pre-PG

ACQUIRED CAUSES OF SNHL

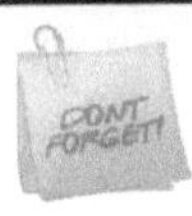 **Sudden Noise TRAUMA**

Sudden – Sudden hearing loss & systemic d/s i.e D.M
Noise – Noise induced hearing loss
T – Trauma to labyrinth or 8th nerve
R - pResbycusis
A – Acoustic neuroma

U – Usual labyrinthine infections
M – Meniere's disease and Multiple sclerosis
A – Alcoholism & smoking

CHARACTERISTICS OF SENSORINEURAL HEARING LOSS

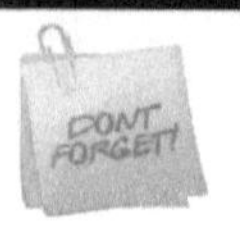

Weber is Not DISABLE

Weber – Weber lateralized to better ear
Not – No gap b/w air & bone conduction curve on audiometry
D – Difficulty in hearing in presence of noise
      I – Involving high frequencies
S – Speech discrimination is poor
A - A positive rinne test AC>BC
B – Bone conduction reduced on schwabach & ABC test
Le – Loss may exceed 60 dB

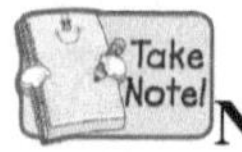

Note – In conductive hearing loss just opposite features

IMPORTANT VIRUSES CAUSING HEARING LOSS

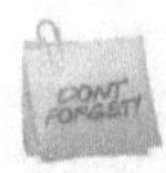

MMR HE

M – Mumps
M - Measles
R - Rubella
HE – Herpes

NON-ORGANIC HEARING LOSS

Either due to malingering or psychogenic
Detected by

REALISTiC tests

R – Reflex test of stapedial
E – Electric response audiometry
A – Absence of shadow curve
L – Lombard's test
I – Inconsistency in PTA & SRT
S – Stenger test
Ti – Teal test
C – Cortical evoked audiometry

EUSTACHIAN TUBE FUNCTION TEST

VaPoRiSaTion
Va – Valsalva test
Po – Politzer test
Ri – Radiological test
Sa – Saccharine & sonotubometry
Ti – Tympanometry & toynbee's
On – Catheterization

OTITIS MEDIA

ASOM

Most common causative organism

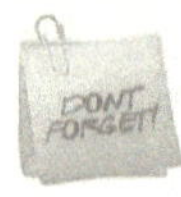

SHM

S – Streptococcus pneumoniae
H -H. influenzae
M – Moraxella catarrhalis

OTOSCOPY SIGNS for ASOM

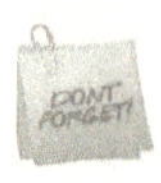

CoLCaTA IPL

Co - Congestion of pars tensa
L – Loss of landmarks
Ca – Cartwheel appearance
T – Translucency reduced
A – Antero-inferior quadrant perforation (most common)
I – Immobile T.M.
P – Pulsatile otorrhea
L – Light house effect

SEQUELAE OF CHRONIC SECRETORTY OTITS MEDIA

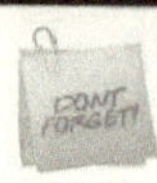

ACTOR

A – Atrophic tympanic membrane & atelectasis of middle ear
C – Cholesterol granuloma
T – Tympanosclerosis
O – Ossicular necrosis
R - Retraction pocket and cholesteotoma

OTOSCOPIC FINDING OF SEROUS OTITIS MEDIA

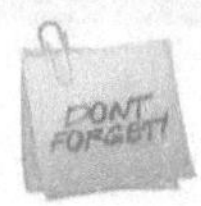

Dull Colour Eardrum due to Bubble Fluid

Dull – Dullness of eardrum
Colour – Colour of eardrum (yellow grey or bluish)
Eardrum – Eardrum retracted with reduced mobility
Bubble – Air bubbles
Fluid– Fluid behind ear drum

CLINICAL FEATURES (C/F) OF CSOM

TUBOTYMPANIC DISEASE

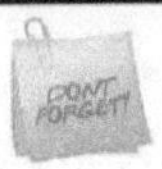

CORN

C – Conductive hearing loss (later may be mixed)
O – Ossicular chain mostly uninvolved (if involved only long process of incus)
R – Round window shielding effect
N – Non-foul-smelling discharge

CLINICAL FEATURES (C/F) OF CSOM

ATTICOANTRAL –

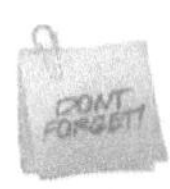

PSBH

P –Posterior marginal perforation of T.M

S – Scanty, foul smelling discharge
B – Bleeding
H – Hearing loss conductive (later may be mixed)

COMPLICATION OF CSOM

PEM* Found in LO Birth

P – Petrositis
E - Extradural abscess
M – Mastoiditis & meningitis
F – Facial paralysis
L- Lateral sinus thrombophlebitis & labyrinthitis
O – Ottic hydrocephalus
B – Brain abscess
S – Subdural abscess

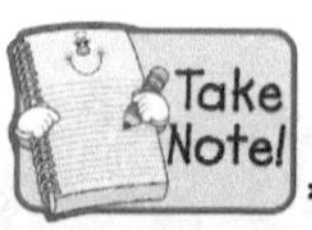

** PEM - protein energy malnutrition*

ATTICOANTRAL DISEASE IS ASSOCIATED

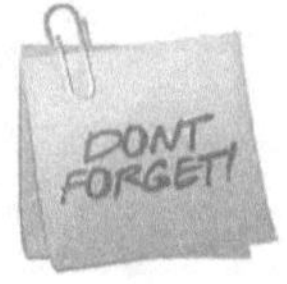

NPCB*

N – Necrosis of ossicle (most common long process of incus)
C – Cholesteatoma & cholesterol granuloma
P – Polyp & granulation tissue
B – Bone destruction & osteitis

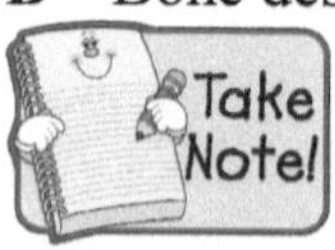

**NPCB – national programme for control of blindness*

ACUTE MASTOIDITIS CLINICAL FEATURES

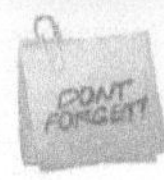

I LOST My Hearing Due To Fever & pain

I – Ironed out skin over mastoid (1st sign)
L – Light house effect
O – Obliteration of retro auricular sulcus
S – Swelling over mastoid pushes pinna forward & downward
S – Tenderness over mastoid
My – Meatal wall sagging
Hearing – Hearing loss conductive
Due - Discharge from ear
To – T.M perforation
Fever
Pain – Pain at MacEvens triangle

GRADENIGO'S SYNROME

TRIAD - DEEP

D – Deep seated orbital or retro orbital pain
E - External rectus palsy
EP – Ear discharge persistent

BELL'S PALSY

It is a Commonest cause of Facial paralysis

Clinical features

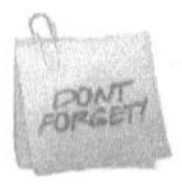

IMPOSIBLE

I – Ipsilateral facial paralysis
M – Most patients recover within few weeks to few month
P – Pt is unable to close his eyes
O – Onset is preceded by pain behind the ear
S – Saliva dribbles from angle of mouth
I – Ipsilateral loss of taste sensation, salivation &lacrimation
B – Bell's phenomenon
L – Loud sound intolerance (hyperacusis)
E – Epiphora

LATERAL SINUS THROMBOPHLEBITIS

Clinical features

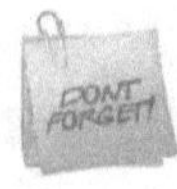

Ten Crow Said Hello to Hectic Green Parrot

Ten- Tenderness along jugular vein
Crow – Crowe –beck test
Said – Severe progressive anaemia
Hello – Headache
TO – Tobey-ayer test
Hectic – Hectic – picket fence type fever with rigor
Green – Griesinger's sign
Parrot – Papilledema

COMPLICATION OF FACIAL PARALYSIS

ICTC *For psychological support

I – Incomplete recovery
C – Crocodile tears & keratitis
T – Tics and spasm
C - Contractures
For – Frey's syndrome
Psychological - Psychological & social problem
Support – Synkinesis

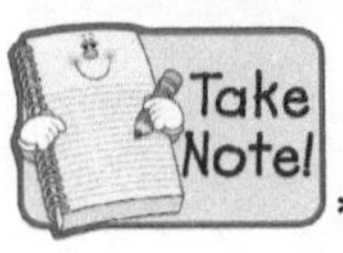

ICTC – integrated counseling & training center

OTOSCLEROSIS & MENIERES DISEASE

MENIERE'S DISEASE

Features of Meniere's d/s

TVS features

T - Tinnitus
V - Vertigo
S – Sensori-neural hearing loss
Feature – Fullness in ear

SIGNS AND SYMPTOMS OF OTOSCLEROSIS SYNROME

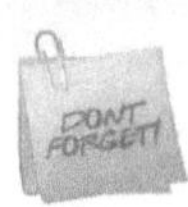

LOSS OF STAPES

Loss of – Loss of hearing & stapedial reflex
S– Speech monotonous
T- Tinnitus
A – 'As 'type tympanogram & acoustic deep 2000 Hz
P – Paracusis willisi
E – vErtigo uncommon
S - Schwartz sign

ETIOLOGY OF MENIERE'S DISEASE

DeVDAS HE

De – Defective absorption by endolymphatic sac
V D- Vasomotor disturbance & viral infection
A – Allergic (50%) & autoimmune
S - Sodium water retention
H – Hypothyroidism

EXAMINATION AND INVESTIGATION OF MENIERE'S DISEASE SYNROME

EXAMINATION – ENT

E – Earscopy(otoscopy) normal T.M.
N - Nystagmus (only during acute attack)
T – Tuning fork test (features of SNHL found)

INVESTIGATION

Girl in SPECS

Girl – Glycerol test (improvement in hearing)
S - Speech audiometry
P - Pure tone audiometry

CONSERVATIVE SURGICAL PROCEDURE FOR MENIERE'S DISEASE

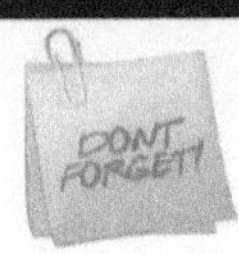

VASUDEV G

Va – Vestibular neuronectomy
S – Dacculotomy (Cody's tack operation) & stellate ganglion block
U – Ultrasonic destruction of vestibular labyrinth
D– Decompression of endolymphatic sac
  E- Endolymphatic shunt operation
V – Vestibular nerve section
G – Gentamycin intratympanic

MEDICAL TREATMENT OF MENIERE'S DISEASE

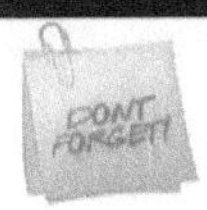

Vada

V – Vasodilator
A – Antihistaminic labyrinthine sedative
D - Diuretics
A – Anxiolytic & tranquillizers

DIFFERENTIAL DIAGNOSIS OF MENIERE'S DISEASE SYNROME

S - Serous otitis media
E – Eustachian tube obstruction
V – Vertebrobasilar insufficiency & migraine
A - Acoustic neuroma
Pe – Perilymph fistula
 O – Occluded auditory canal by wax
P – Paget's d/s
L - Labyrinthitis
E - Endocrine(hypothyroidism)

SUBJECTIVE CAUSES OF TINNITUS

OTOLOGIC

MOTA Wax Pressing ET or Nerve

Me – Meniere's d/s
O – Ototoxic drugs, Otosclerosis
T – Trauma (noise)
A – Acute & chronic otitis media
Wax - Impacted wax
Pressing - Presbycusis
E T - Abnormally patent Eustachian Tube
N – Tumour of 8th nerve

NON-OTOLOGIC

ADMI HE *2

A - Arteriosclerosis
A - Anemia
D - D/s of CNS
D - Drugs
Mi - Migraine
He- Hypo & hypertension
He – Hypoglycemia

CLINICAL FFEATURE OF ACOUSTIC NEUROMA

When confined to internal auditory canal

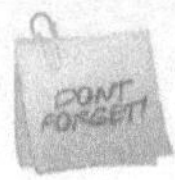

IUD

I – Imbalance (true vertigo is rare)
U –Unilateral sensorineural deafness/tinnitus
D –Difficulty in understanding speech *

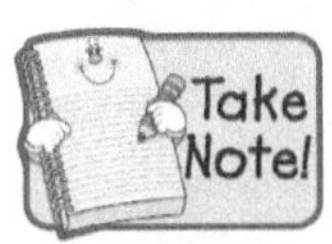

(*characteristic feature)

TUMOR INVESTIGATIONS OF ACOUSTIC NEUROMA

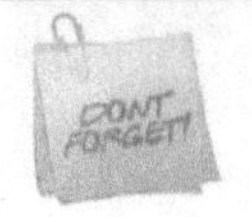

STAR Ca speech score

S – SNHL is more marked in high frequencies
T– Tone decay is significant
A – Acoustic reflex
R – Recruitment absent
Ca – Caloric test (diminished or absent)

Speech – Speech discrimination is highly impaired
Score – SISI score 0-20%

NASAL GLIOMA

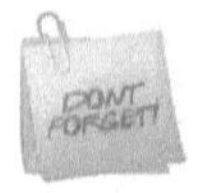

Features –NOR FLOX

N – Non-tender
O - Overlying skin red, bluish or telangiectatic
R – Route of nose par
F - Firm
Lo - Located to one side
X - Xpand not on crying or pulsate

INVERTED PAPILLOMA

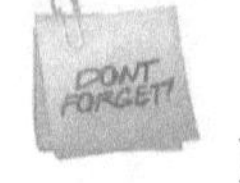

Features – unilateral NASAL obstruction

unilateral - unilateral always & cause unilateral epistaxis
N – Nose runny
A – Aggressive locally
S – Squamous carcinoma se associated
A – Adequate local excision is t/t
L – Lateral wall of nose se arises
Obstruction - Obstruction of nose occur

CLINICAL FEATURES OF NASOPHARYNGEAL CARCINOMA

In order of frequency

CHaNE

C – Cervical lymphadenopathy
Ha – Hearing loss
N - Nasal obstruction
E – Epistaxis

CLINICAL FEATURES OF GLOMUS TUMOR

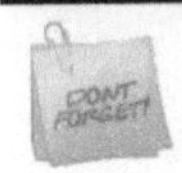

PAPPu Sala FAIL He

P – Pulsatile tinnitus (earliest symptom)
A – Aquino sign
P – Polyp will be seen (when tumor perforate eardrum)
Pu – Pulsation sign (brown sign)
Sala - Sun rising appearance
F - Facial palsy may be caused by glomus tympanicum
A – Audible systolic bruit
I – Increased catecholamine secretion
L – Late cranial nerve palsies
He – Hearing loss

JUVENILE NASOPHARYNGEAL ANGIOFIBROMA

SANAM BEVFA (movie name)

S – Spontaneous profuse & recurrent epistaxis
A – Antral sign (Holman-miller sign)
Na - Nasal obstruction (most common symptom)
M – Margin of sphenopalatine foramen is most common site
B – Benign & bilobed
E – Exclusively in male
V – Vessels are just endothelial lined
F – Frog-face deformity
A – Adolescent (7-19) me common

OSSEUS PART OF NASAL SEPTUM

VERNA Fluidic (Hyundai car)

V - Vomer
E – Ethmoid
R – Rostrum & crest of sphenoid
Na– Nasal crest of palatine, maxillary ,& nasal bone
F – Frontal bone nasal spine

NASAL SEPTUM CAUSES OF SEPTAL PERFORATION

PERFORATION

P – Poisons (cocaine, topical steroid, decongestant)
E – E(i)nflammation chronic (wegner's, T.B., syphilis, leprosy, sarcoidosis,atrophic rhinitis)
R – Rhinolith
FOR – FOReign body
A – As a complication of septal abscess
T –Trauma (m.c.c) & tumors of septum
I - Idiopathic
O – Operational procedure of nose
N – Nasal myiasis

CLINICAL FEATURES OF DNS

NASAL Deformity HE

Na - Nasal obstruction
S – Sinusitis
A - Anosmia

L – midd**L**e ear infection
Deformity – Deformity of external nose
H – Headache
E – Epistaxis

CHOANAL ATRESIA

Bilateral cases in 20-30% pt, 50% of these Associated with

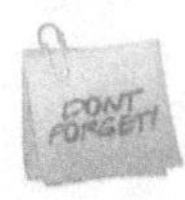

CHARGE syndrome

C - Coloboma
H – Heart defect
A – Atresia of choana
R – Retarded growth
G – Genitourinary
E – Ear defects

4 ARTERIES CONTRIBUTE TOO LITTLE'S AREA

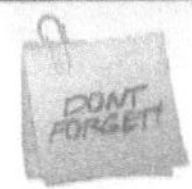

GAS

G – Greater palatine
A – Ant. Ethmoidal
S- Septal branch of superior labial and sphenopalatine

LOCAL CAUSES OF EPISTAXIS IN NOSE –

BAD Trauma In Nose

B – Bodies (foreign bodies living & nonliving)
A – atmospheric changes
D - DNS

Trauma - trauma
In- infection (acute & chronic)
Nose– neoplasm of nose & paranasal sinuses)

IN NASOPHARYNX -

JAM

J - Juvenile angiofibroma
A – Adenoiditis
M – Malignant tumor

RHINITIS & SINUSITIS

CAUSES OF RECURRENT EPISTAXIS IN CHILDREN

RIHANA

R – Retained nasal foreign bodies
I – Intranasal sprays
H – Hemorrhagic disease as ITP
A - Angiofibroma
N – Nasal myiasis & parasitosis
A – Allergic rhinitis

RHINITIS

PRIMARY ATROPHIC RHINITIS CAUSES

HERNIA

H - Hereditary

E – Endocrine disturbance
R – Racial factor
N – Nutritional deficiency
I - Infective
A – Autoimmune process

CLINICAL FEATURES OF ATROPHIC RHINITIS

AFMC HE
A - Always bilateral
F - Foul smell & female(common)
M – Marked anosmia
C – Crust filling the nose
H – Hoarseness may occur
E – Epistaxis
Surgical t/t – YaMLa – Young's operation modified young's operation, Lautenslagers operation

ACUTE SINUSITIS

Most common bacteria

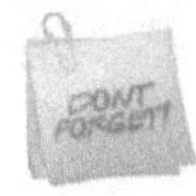

SHM
S – Streptococcus pneumoniae
H – H. influenzae
M – Moraxella catarrhalis

TYPES OF CHRONIC RHINITIS

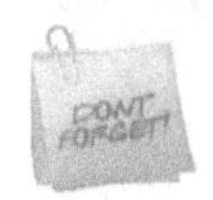

CHAR
C – Chronic simple rhinitis

H - Hypertrophic
A - Atrophic
R – Rhinitis sicca & caseosa

ETIOLOGY OF SINUSITIS

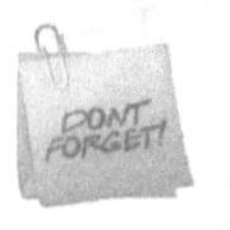

Exciting factors - Nasal STD

Nasal – Nasal infection
S – Swimming & diving
T - Trauma
D – Dental infection

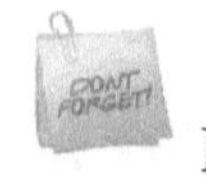

Predisposing factors- SAD

S–Stasis of secretion in nose
A- Allergies
D – Drainage & ventilation of sinus obstructed

CLINICAL FEATURES of ACUTE SINUSITIS

MAJOR

FUND oF

Fu–Fullness of face, pain
N – Nasal obstruction
D – Discharging nose
Of -Fever

MINOR

HDFCe

H - Halitosis & headache
D – Dental pain congestion
F – Fatigue
C – Cough
E – Ear pain

LOCAL & ORBITAL COMPLICATION OF CHRONIC SINUSITIS

MOM Ca SOOP

LOCAL

MOM

M - Mucocele
O - Osteomyelitis
M - Mucus retention cyst

ORBITAL

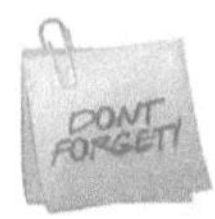

CA SOOP

CA - Cavernous sinus thrombosis
S – Superior orbital fissure syndrome & subperiosteal abscess
O – Orbital cellulitis & abscess
O – Orbital apex syndrome
P – Periorbital cellulitis & neuritis

CHRONIC SINUSITIS

Clinical Features

Sour Taste in Throat during Swallowing

Sour – Sore throat attacks acute tonsillitis
Taste – Bad taste in mouth & foul breath
Throat – Throat irritation with cough
Swallowing – Swallowing difficulty and choking

EXAMINATION -

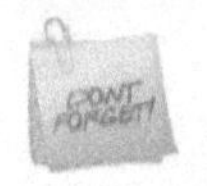

Yellow CoFE

Yellow - Yellow beads of pus on medial surface of tonsil
Co – Congestion of anterior pillars
F – Frank pus or cheesy material on pressure
E – Enlargement of jugulodigastric lymph nodes

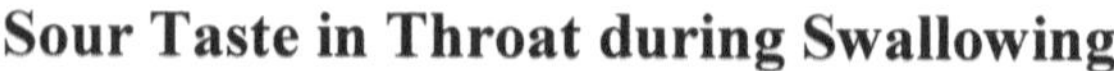

SYMPTOMS OF ETHMOIDAL POLYPI

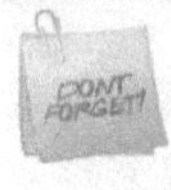

DiL He ki Manta Nahi

Di – Discharge from nose &sneezing
L – Loss of sense of smell
He - Headache
Manta- Mass protruding from nostril
Nahi - Nasal stuffiness

TYPES OF FUNGAL SINUSITIS

FAFundI

F – Fungal ball
A – Allergic fungal sinusitis
Fu – **Fu**lminant fungal sinusitis
I – Invasive sinusitis (chronic)

CLINICAL FEATURES OF ZYGOMATIC FRACTURE (tripod fracture)

FRACTURES

F – Flattening of malar prominence
R - Restricted ocular movement (cause diplopia)
A - Anesthesia in distribution of infraorbital nerve
C – Considerable swelling over zygomatic arch
T - Trismus
U–obliq**U**e palpebral fissure
R – pe**R**iorbital emphysema
E - Epistaxis
S – Step deformity of infraorbital margin

CLINICAL FEATURES OF MAXILLARY FRACTURE

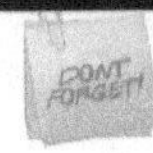

I aM CM

I – Injury to infraorbital nerve In Le fort II & III fracture
aM - Malocclusion of teeth
C – CSF rhinorrhea (II &III Fracture)
M – Mobility in maxilla

DETECTION OF CSF LEAK

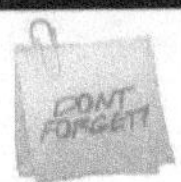

Quick RFT for increase glucose & B2 transferrin

Quick – Queckensted test
R- Rhinoscopy
F – Filter paper test (halo sign)
T – Tissue test (handkerchief test)
 Increase – Intrathecal fluorescene dye administration
Glucose – Glucose is higher in CSF
B2 transferrin (definitive test)

ADENOID FACIES

Symptoms –

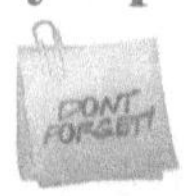

HOTEL
H – High arched palate & hitched upper lip
O – Open mouth
T – Teeth are overcrowded & prominent
E – Elongated face
L – Lack of concentration(aprosexia)

PHARYNX

Symptoms of acute tonsillitis

Can't Swallow Sour Fruit Ever

Can't – Constitutional symptoms (headache, body ache, malaise)
Swallowing – Swallowing difficulty
Sour - Sore throat
Fever - Fever with chills & rigors
Ever- Earache

DIFFERENTIAL DIAGNOSIS OF MEMBRANE OVER TONSIL

MEDICAL TrauMA

M – Membranous tonsillitis
E - Ephthus ulcer
D - Diphtheria
I - Infectious mononucleosis
C - Candidiasis
A – Agranulocytosis & angina (Vincent's)
L - Leukemia
Trau – Traumatic ulcer
Ma - Malignancy tonsil

LARYNX

CLINICAL FEATUES OF PERITONSILLAR ABSCESS

LOCAL –

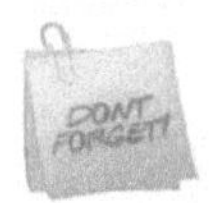

SOFTI voice

S – Severe pain in throat
O - Odynophagia
F – Foul breath
T - Trismus
I – Ipsilateral earache
Voice – Hot potato voice

MUSCLES OF LARYNX

INTRINSIC MUSCLES

PoLaTICs for VOTING

Po – Posterior cricoarytenoid (abductors)
La – Lateral cricoarytenoid
T - Thyroarytenoid
I - Interarytenoid
C- Cricothyroid
V – Vocalis
O – Oblique part of interarytenoid (post.)
T - Thyroepiglotic
Ing - Interarytenoid

EPIGLOTTITIS

Very tasty dinner in CCD

Very – Vallecula sign
Tasty – Thumb sign
Dinner – Drooling of saliva
In - Influenza (most common cause) inspiratory retraction
C - Cyanosis
C – Cherry red and swollen epiglottis
D – Dysphagia

CONTACT GRANULOMA (CONTACT ULCER)

VIP HE INDIA Bhi

V – Vocal abuse is primary cause
I – Intubation is primary cause
P – Posterior third of vocal cord site common
H – Hoarseness or husky voice
E – Esophageal reflex (GERD) is primary cause

I – Idiopathic causes
N – Neoplastic change does not occur
D - Discomfort
I - Irritation
A – Acanthosis
B – Biopsy necessary to differentiate it from T.B. & carcinoma
Hi – hyperkeratosis

LARYNGOTRACHEOBRONCHITIS (CROUP)

Presentation -

CROUPS

C - Croupy cough (barking cough) & hoarseness
R – Respiratory stridor
O – Oedema in subglottic area
U – Upper airway obstruction sign
P - Parainfluenza virus (most frequently)
S – Steeple sign (narrowing of subglottic region) in x-ray

T.B. LARYNGITIS

Laryngeal examination

PSM Is Tuff Subject to Memorize

P – Post. Part or whole of vocal cord is hyperemic
S – Swelling of ventricular bands and aryepiglottic folds
M – Mouse-nibbled appearance of vocal cord
Is – Interarytenoid region, granulation tissue present
Tuff - Turban epiglottis (pseudo edema of epiglottis)
Subject – Superficial ragged ulceration on arytenoids & interarytenoid region
Memorize - Mamillated appearance

SQUAMOUS PAPILOMA OF LARYNX

JUVENILE PAPILOMA

IMP. FEATURES –

HUMAN

H – Human papilloma virus or common cause HPV6& 11
U – Usual features are hoarseness & cry under 5 yr of age
M – Multiple recurrent papilloma in larynx
A - Associated with maternal genital wart
N– Not malignant but prone to malignant

PLUMMER – VINSON *SYNDROME*

DIALOGuE

D - Dysphagia
I – Iron deficiency anemia
A – Angular stomatitis
L - koiLonychia
Gu - Glossitis
E – Esophageal web

PREMALIGNANT CONDITION OF LARYNX

MEDIKAL HE

M – Microinvasive carcinoma
E - Erythroplakia
D - Dysplasia

I - In situ carcinoma
KA – Keratosis with Atypia
L – Leukoplakia & laryngeal papilloma (juvenile)
He- Hyperplasia

DIAGNOSTIC AND OPERATIVE ENT

INDICATION OF MYRINGOTOMY

Aasa
A – ASOM (with CBI, C – Complication, B – bulging T.M., I – incomplete resolution)
A - Aero O.M
S - SOM
A – Atelectatic ear

TYPES OF TYMPANOPLASTY

My Most common game football
TYPE
My - Myringotomy
  Most – Malleus or incus graft
  Common – Columella operation
  Game – Graft placed b/w oval & round window
 Football - Fenestration operation

GRAFT MATERIAL USED FOR MYRINGOPLASTY

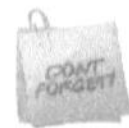

PVT team

P – Perichondrium from tragus
V – Vein
T – Tragal cartilage
Team - Temporalis fascia

INDICATION FOR CORTICAL MASTOIDECTOMY

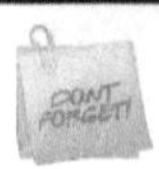

AIMS

A – Acute coalescent mastoiditis
I – Incompletely resoled acute otitis media with reservoir sign
M – Masked mastoiditis
S – Step to perform - endolymphatic sac surgery
decompression of facial nerve
trans or retro labyrinthine procedure

SMR OPERATION

INDICATION

SARA

S–Symptomatic DNS
A – As a part of septorhinoplasty
R - Recurrent epistaxis
A – As a preliminary step in Hypophysectomy

CONTRAINDICATION

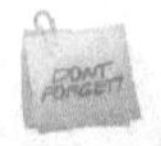

BABU

B – Below 17 yr
A– Acute episode of respiratory infection
B– Bleeding diathesis
U – Untreated D.M. or hypertension

INDICATION OF TONSLLECTOMY

ABSOLUTE

RePeAT Hypertrophy Me

Re –Recurrent infection of throat
PeA – Peritonsillar Abscess
T - Tonsillitis causing febrile seizures
Hypertrophy- of tonsil
Me – Malignancy suspicion

RELATIVE

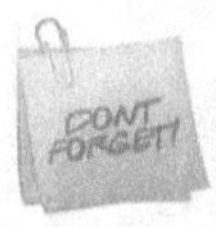

DCR

D – Diphtheria & streptococcal carrier
C – Chronic tonsillitis unresponsive to medical treatment
R – Recurrent streptococcal tonsillitis in valvular heart disease

INDICATION OF FESS

ENDOSCOPIC Septoplasty

E – Ethmoid & antral polyp
N – Nose bleeding (epistaxis)
D – Decompression of optic nerve
O – Orbital decompression for GRAVE's d/s
S – Sinus mucocele
C – Chronic bacterial sinusitis
O – Orbital abscess & cellulitis
P – Polypoid rhinosinusitis & nasal polypi
I – Inverted papilloma & other benign tumor
C – Choanal atresia

Septoplasty – Endoscopic septoplasty

CONTRAINDICATTION OF TONSILLECTOMY

BAChHO ME under 3 yr

B – Bleeding disorder
A – Acute upper respiratory tract infection me
Ch – Child < 3 yr
H – Hb < 10 g%
O – Overt or submucous soft palate
M – Menses period
E – Epidemic of polio
Under 3 yr - Uncontrolled systemic disease

IN INDIRECT LARYNGOSCOPY FOLLOWING AR

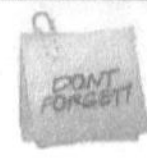

SIVA

S – Subglottic area
I – Infrahyoid epiglottis
V - Ventricles
A - Anterior commissure

TYPES OF TRACHEOSTOMY

Emergency ill pt per mini tracheostomy (karte he)

Emergency - Emergency tracheostomy
ill - ELECTIVE
pt - Permanent
per – Percutaneous
mini – Tracheostomy

INDICATION OF CALDWELL-LUC OPERATION

 **CRVO DRAIN karne ke liye**

C – Chronic maxillary sinusitis with irreversible change in mucosa
R –Recurrent antrochoanal polyp
V – Vidian neurectomy
O – Oroantral fistula
D – Dental cyst
R – removal of foreign body or route of tooth
A – As an approach to ethmoids & pterygopalatine fossa
I - In blow out fracture or maxillary fracture
N – Neoplasm (suspected)

INDICATION OF TRACHEOSTOMY

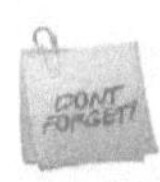 **BRONChI Trauma OF PAI**

B – Bilateral abductor paralysis
R – foReign body
O – Oedema larynx
N - Neoplasm
Ch - Congenital anamolies
I - Infection
Trauma OF
P – Painful cough
A – Aspiration of pharyngeal secretion
I – Inability to cough& insufficiency of respiratory system

INDICATION OF ADENOIDECTOMY

 **RADAR**

R – Recurrent rhinosinusitis

A – Adenoid hypertrophy (causing symptoms)
D – Dental malocclusion
A – Adenoid hyperplasia associated   with chronic secretory otitis media
R – Recurrent ear discharge in CSOM a/w adenoiditis/adenoid hyperplasia

INDICATION OF ADENOIDECTOMY

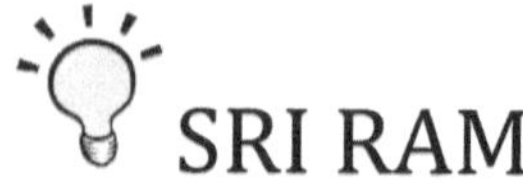 SRI RAM

S – Side effect of topical drugs
R – Retinal vascular disorder
I – Intraocular inflammations & tumor
R –Retinal dystrophies
A – As post-operative complication
M – Macular traction (vitreo) & macular epiretinal membrane

SIGNS OF BACTERIAL CORNEA ULCER

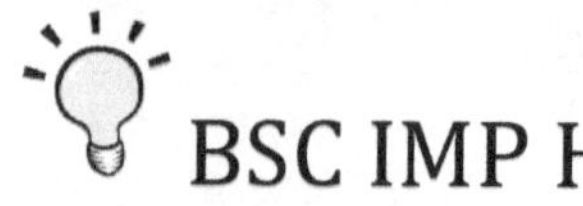 BSC IMP Hy

B - Blepharospasm
S – Swelling of lid
C – Corneal ulcer, Cornea chemosed and Hyperemia
I – Intraocular pressure raised
M – Muddy iris
P – Pupil small
Hy – Hypopyon

EARLY OPERATIVE COMPLICATION

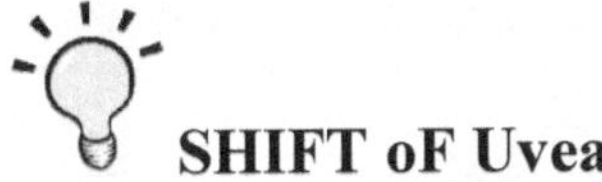 **SHIFT oF Uvea**

S – Striate keratopathy
H - Hyphaema
I– Iris prolapse
F – Flate ant. chamber
T – Toxic anterior segment syndrome
oF – oFthalmitis (endophthalmitis)
Uvea – Uveitis (anterior)

LATE POSTOPERATIVE COMPLICATION

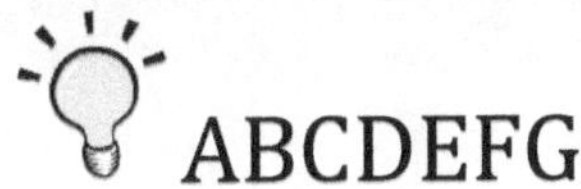 ABCDEFG

A –After cataract
B – Bullous keratopathy (pseudophakic)
C– Cystoid macular edema
D – Detachment of retina and delay endophthalmitis
E- Epithelial ingrowth
F– Fibrous downgrowth
G – Glaucoma

OPERATIVE COMPLICATION OF CATARACT SURGERY

 **DEEP INCISION**

D– Dehiscence of zonula
E– Excessive bleeding
E - Expulsive choroidal hemorrhage
P – Posterior Capsular rupture

I – Iris injury and iridodialysis
N – Nucleus drop
C – Complication related to anterior capsulorrhexis
I – Incision related complication
S – Superior Rectus muscle laceration
I – Injury to cornea
O – lOss of vitreous
N - leNs fragments loss

IOL RELATED COMPLICATION

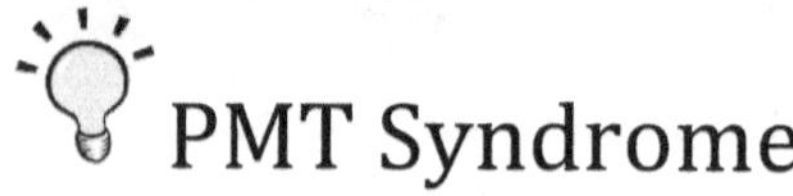 PMT Syndrome

P – Pupillary capture of IOL
M – Malposition of IOL
T – Toxic anterior segment syndrome
Syndrome – UGH syndrome

EARLY GLAUCOMATOUS CHANGES

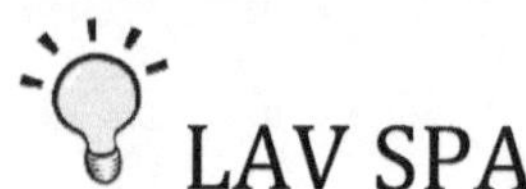 LAV SPA

L – Large cup >0.6
A – Asymmetry of cup
V – Vertical oval cup
S – Splinter hemorrhage
P – Pallor areas
A – Atrophy of retinal nerve

INVESTIGATION OF GLAUCOMA

 **C T DSP GONE**

C – Central corneal thickness
T - Tonometry
D – Diurnal variation
S - Slit lamp examination
P – Perimetry and provocative test (water drinking)
Go - Gonioscopy
Ne – Nerve fiber layer analyzer

ADVANCE GLAUCOMATOUS CHANGES

 **ThaNa Ma Pandey on Duty**

Tha – Thinning of neuroretinal rim
Na – Nasal shifting of retinal vessel
Ma - Marked cupping 0.7-0.9
Pandey – Pulsation of retinal arteriole
On
Duty- Dot sign(lamellar)

LAYERS OF RETINA

From without inward

Pigment layer after that L M N O P

L – Layer of rods and cones
M - Membrane (external limiting)
N – Nuclear layer (outer)
OP - Outer plexiform layer

OPHTHALMOSCOPIC PICTURE OF NON-PROLIFERATIVE DIABETIC RETINOPATHY

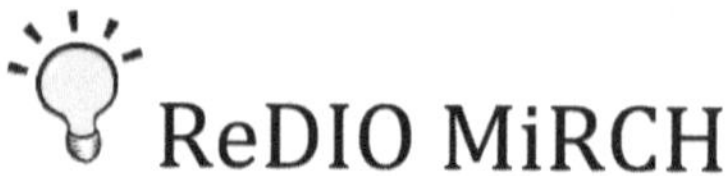 ReDIO MiRCH

Re – Retinal hemorrhages
D – Dark-blot hemorrhages
I – IRMA (intra-retinal microvascular abnormalities)
O - Oedema
Mi - Microaneurysm
R - abno**R**malities
C – Cotton wool spot
H – Hard exudate

PERIPHERAL RETINAL DEGENERATION

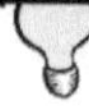 White FOCAL Degeneration

White – White with pressure & without
Fo – Focal pigment clump
C – Chorioretinal & cystoid retinal
A – Acquired retinoschisis
L - Lattice

Degeneration - Snail track **Degeneration**

OPHTHALMOSCOPIC FEATURES OF PAPILLEDEMA

 BADMaS COMPNE He

Early papilledema –

B – Blurring of peripapillary nerve fiber layer
A – Absence of spontaneous venous pulsation
D – Disc margin obscuration
Ma – Mild hyperemia of disc
S – Splinter hemorrhage

Established

C – Circumferential greyish white fold in disc
O – Obliterated cup
M – Multiple cotton wool spot
P – forward elevation above the **P**lane of retina
N – Ngorged & Tortuous vein
E - Exudate(hard)

DIFFERENTIAL DIAGNOSIS OF LEUKOCORIA

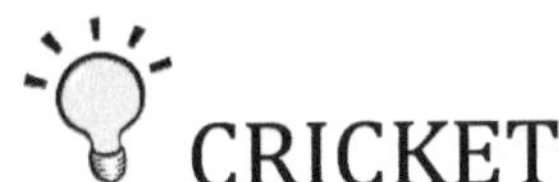 CRICKET

C – Congenital cataract
R – Retrolental fibroplasia
I – Inflammatory deposit in vitreous & Vitreous hyperplasia
CK - Coloboma of koroid
E – Exudative retinopathy of Coats
T – Toxocara endophthalmitis

TYPES OF VERNAL KERATOPATHY

 UPSC

U – Ulcerative
P – Punctate & Pseudogerontoxon
S – Subepithelial Scarring
C - Cornel Plaques

TYPES OF BLEPHARITIS

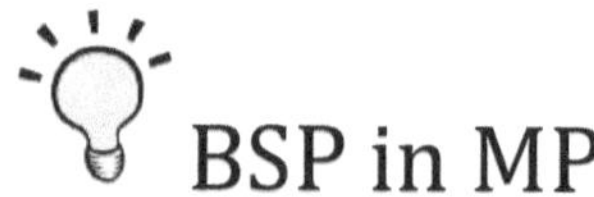 BSP in MP

B - Bacterial
S - Seborrheic
P- Parasitic
In
M – Mixed Staphylococcal
P – Posterior Blepharitis

CORNEAL SIGNS OF VERNAL KERATOPATHY

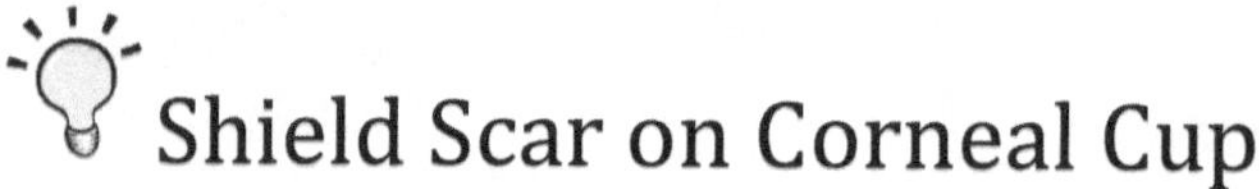 Shield Scar on Corneal Cup

Shield - Shield Ulcer
Scar - Subepithelial Scarring
Corneal- Corneal plaques
Cup - Cupids bowretinal

CAUSES OF AXIAL MYOPIA

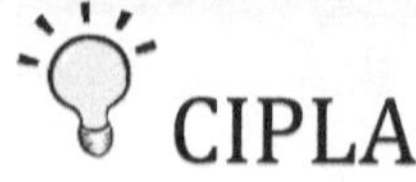 CIPLA

C - Curvatural

I - Index
P - Positional
L – Lens (absent)
A – Axial

LAYERS OF CORNEA

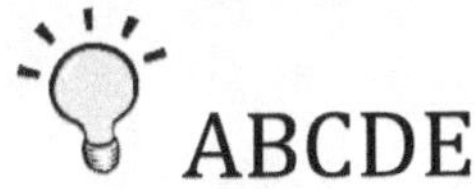 ABCDE

A - Apithelium
B - Bowman's
C – Corneal Stroma
D - Descemet's
E – Endothelium

TREATMENT OF INTERMEDIATE UVEITIS (KAPLAN protocol)

S – Systemic Steroid
I – Immunosuppressive drugs
L – Laser Photocoagulation (indirect)
Pa – Pars-plana Vitrectomy

DRUG CAUSING COLORED HALOS

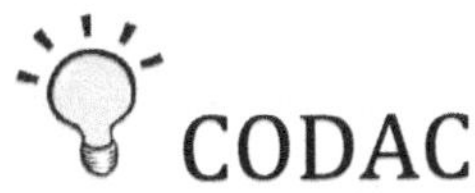 CODAC

C- Cortisone, Chloroquine
O - OCP
D-Digoxin
A-Amiodarone

C-Chlorpromazine

1.73 CHOROIDAL NEOVASCULARIZATION IS ASSOCIATED WITH

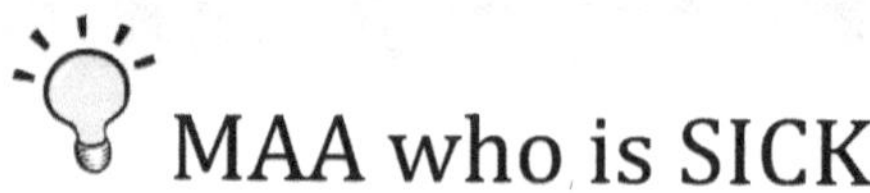 MAA who is SICK

M –Myopia (pathological)
A - ARMD
A – Angioid Streak
who is
S – Scar Chorioretinal
I – Intraocular inflammation
C – Chorioretinal dystrophy
K – Koroidal rupture

1.49 CAUSES OF KERATOCONUS

Systemic

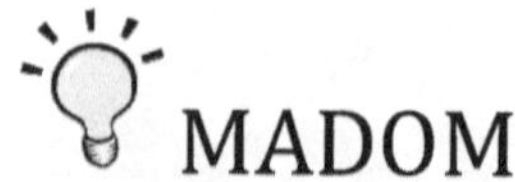 MADOM

M- Marfan syndrome
A- Atopy (Asthma, Eczema, Atopic Keratoconjunctivitis, Hay fever)
D- Danlos syndrome and down syndrome
O- Osteogenesis Imperfecta
M-Mitral Valve Prolapse

1.66 CAUSES OF ENLARGED CORNEAL NERVE

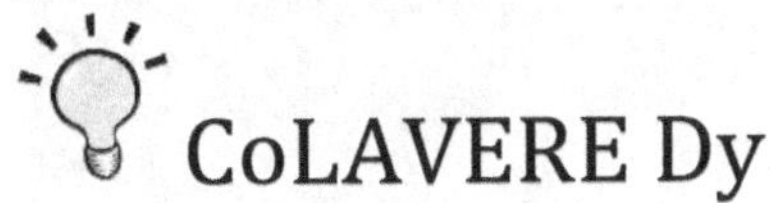

Mujhe Tumse Kuch KAHNA he GIRL Frnd

Mujhe – MEN 2b
Tumse - Trauma
Kuch - Keratoconus
K– Keratoconjunctivitis sicca
A – Acanthamoeba keratitis
H – Hereditary ectodermal dysplasia
N – Neurofibromatosis
A he - Advance age
G – Glaucoma (congenital)
I - Ichthyosis
R – Refsum's disease
L- Leprosy
Frnd – Fuch's dystrophy and failed Corneal graft

OCULAR CAUSES OF KERATOCONUS

CoLAVERE Dy

Co - Congenital Cataract
L- Leber's congenital amaurosis
A-Aniridia
V-Vernal Conjunctivitis
E-Ectopia Lentis
R - Retinitis Pigmentosa
E-Eyelid Syndrome(floppy)
Dy-Dystrophy

1.50 CAUSES OF CORNEAL VASCULARIZATION

Superficial

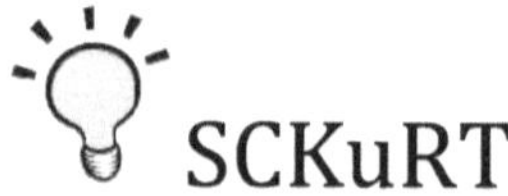 **SCKuRT**

S - Superficial Corneal ulcer
C - Contact lens user
Ku- Keratoconjunctivitis (phlyctenular)
R- Rosacea Keratitis
T- Trachoma

Deep

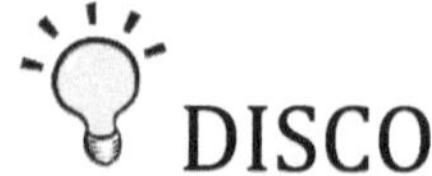 **DISCO**

D - Disciform keratitis and deep corneal ulcer
I – Interstitial keratitis
S – Sclerosing keratitis
Co – Corneal graft rejection and chemical burn

1.66 DRUG CAUSES PIGMENT DEPOSITION IN CORNEA

 **TINA Causes Colorful Cornea**

T - Tilorone
I - Indomethacin
N - Naproxen
A - Amiodarone
Causes- Chloroquine
Colorful - Clofazimine
Cornea – Chlorpromazine

SYSTEMIC D/S CAUSES CATARACT

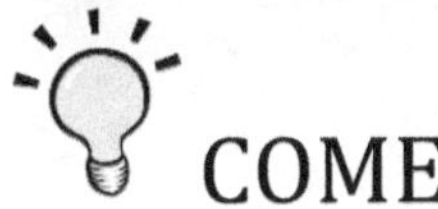 Pouch of DAGLAS Hy

Pouch – Parathyroidism(hypo)
D – Dystrophia Myotonica, DM, Down Syndrome
A – Alport Syndrome
G – Galactosemia, galactokinase deficiency
L – Lowe syndrome
S – Stickler syndrome
Hy – Hypertension, Hypothyroidism

1.67 CAUSES OF BLUE SCLERA

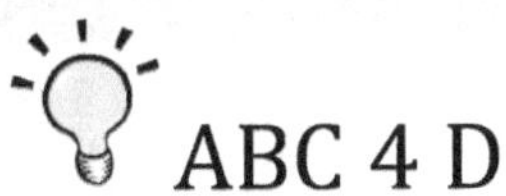 COME

C –Congenital Glaucoma
O – Osteogenesis Imperfecta
M - Marfan syndrome
E – Ehrler Danlos syndrome and elasticum pseudoxanthoma

TOXIC AGENT CAUSES CATARACT

ABC 4 D

A - Amiodarone, Anticholinesterase
B - Busulfan
C - Corticosteroid, Chloroquine, Cigarette, Chlorpromazine
D – Diuretics

1.85 TYPES OF CONGENITAL CATARACT

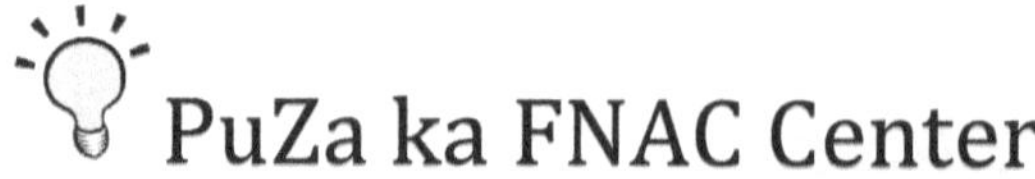 PuZa ka FNAC Center

Pu – Punctate cataract
Za – Zonular cataract
F – Fusiform
N - Nuclear
A – Anterior Capsular
C - Coronary
C – Capsular (post)

1.93 CAUSES OF ECTOPIA LENTIS

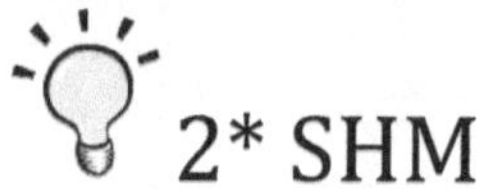 2* SHM

S – Sulphite oxidase deficiency
S - Stickler Syndrome
H – Homocystinuria
H - Hyperlysinemia
M – Marfan syndrome
M – Marchesanii–Weil syndrome

CAUSES OF HARD EXUDATE

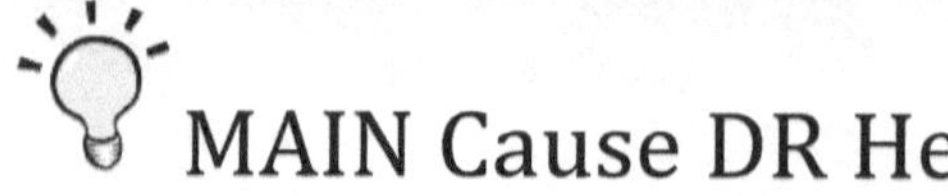 MAIN Cause DR He

M –Microaneurysm, Neovascularization, CRVO
A - Anemia
I – Infection
N - Neoplasm, Leukemia

Cause – Collagen vascular disorder
DR – Diabetic Retinopathy
H – Hypertension
E- Eye disease

CAUSES OF CHERRY RED SPOT

CHERRY RED SPOT KAHA MILTA HE?

Cherry red spot = red lipistic
Ans is- **Girls Common Room Me MiLTa Ha**

G – Gangliosidoses GM1 and GM2
C - CRAO
R – Rarely in krabbe's disease
Me – Metachromatic leukodystrophy
Mi – Multiple sulfates deficiency
L – Lipid storage disorder i.e Niemann-pick, Gaucher
Ta - Trauma
H – Hurler's and Hallervorden disease

RETINAL DETACHMENT

Causes of rhegmatogenous retinal detachment

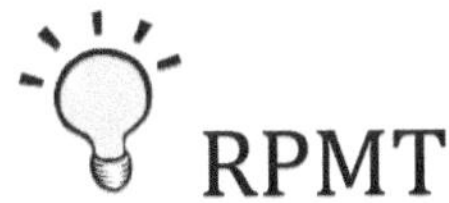 RPMT

R – Retinal degeneration
P - Previous intraocular surgery
M – Myopia
T – Trauma

EXUDATIVE RETINAL DETACHMENT

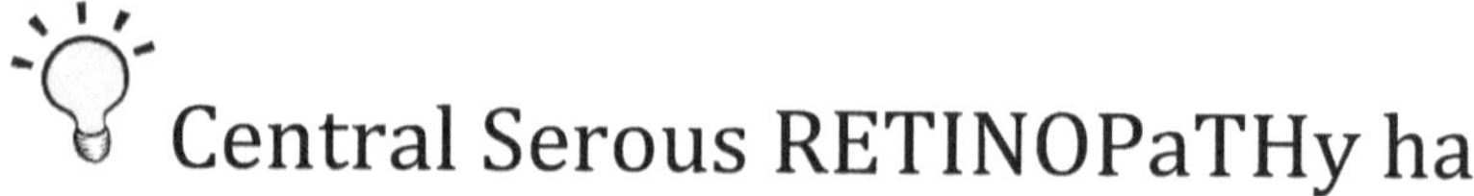 # Central Serous RETINOPaTHy ha

Central – central serous retinopathy
S – Sympathetic ophthalmitis
R – Renal Hypertension
E – Exudative retinopathy of coat's
T – Toxemia of pregnancy
I – Intraocular operation
N – Neovascularization of choroid
O – Orbital cellulitis
Pa – Post. scleritis, pan
T - Tumor of choroid
Hy – Hypertension
Ha – Harada's disease

TRACTIONAL RETINAL DETACHMENT

Let retina = color poster then in detachment

 # Color POSTER Pr Penetration hota he

Color -
Po- Post hemorrhagic retinitis proliference
S – Sickle cell retinopathy
T - Toxocariasis
E – Eale's disease
R – Retinopathy of prematurity
Pr - Proliferative diabetic retinopathy
Penetration – Penetrating injury

SYNDROME A/W RETINITIS PIGMENTOSA

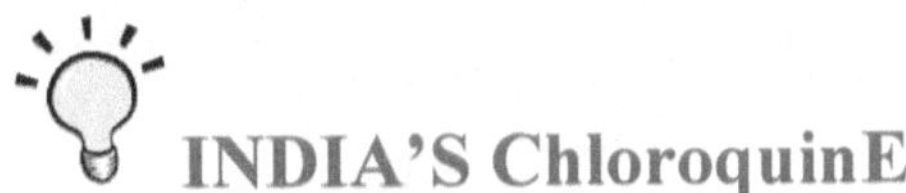

HURLar's BANK syndrome

H - Hallgren's syndrome
U – Usher's syndrome
R – Refsum's syndrome
Lar – Laurence syndrome
S - Cockaynes syndrome
B – Bardet-Biedle syndrome
A – Abetalipoproteinemia (bussen synd.)
N - NARP
K – Kearns-Sayer syndrome

OPTIC NEURITIS

Causes of toxic amblyopia

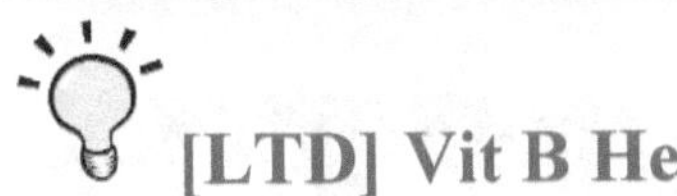

INDIA'S ChloroquinE

I – Isoniazid
N - NSAIDS
D - Digoxin
I – Indica Cannabis
A – Alcohols (ethyl, methyl, glycol), amiodarone
S – Streptomycin
C - Chloroquine
E – Ethambutol

CAUSES OF PRIMARY OPTIC ATROPHY

[LTD] Vit B He

L – Leber's hereditary neuritis
T – Trauma, tabes dorsalis, toxic amblyopia
D – Demyelinating disorder
V - Vit B deficiency
H – Hydrocephalus

CAUSES OF BULL'S EYE MACULOPATHY

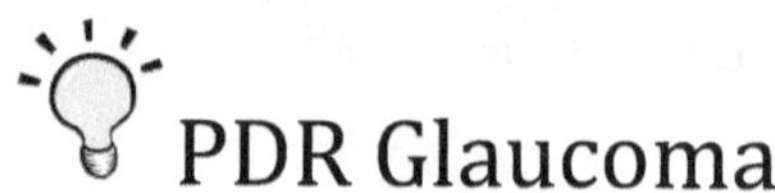 **PCB in ISC boarD padhte padhte bulls eye ho jati he**

P - Phenothiazine
C - Chloroquine
B - Bardet-Biedle syndrome
in **I** - Inverse retinitis pigmentosa
S – Stargardt disease
C – Chronic macular hole
Boar - Batten disease
D - Dystrophies of macula

CAUSES OF CONSECUTIVE OPTIC ATROPHY

PDR Glaucoma

P - Pathological myopia
D – Diffuse chorioretinitis
R – Retinitis pigmentosa
G - Glaucoma and CRAO

TESTS FOR COLOR VISION

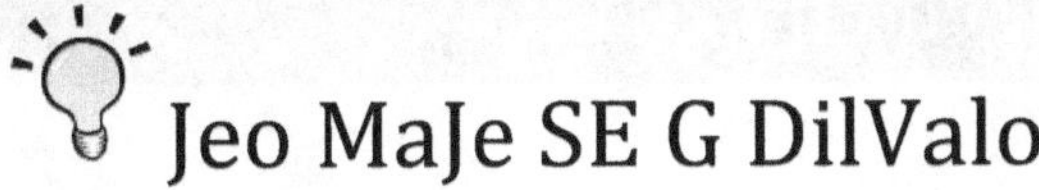 Pseudo Green Wool Test for Nag City

Pseudo - Pseudoisochromatic chart
Green – Green Lantern test
Wool – Holmgreen **Wools** test
Test – Fansworth Munsell test
Nagpur– Nagel's anomaloscope
City – City university test

OCULAR SIGNS IN THYROID OPHTHALMOPATHY

Jeo MaJe SE G DilValo

Jeo –Joffrey's sign
Ma – Mobius sign
Je – Jelinek's sign
S – Stellwag sign
E – Enroth's sign
G –Gifford's sign
Dil – Dalrymple's sign
Valo – Von graefe's sign

All differential diagnosis mentioned above have been asked in Pre
PG exams

INDICATORS OF HEALTH

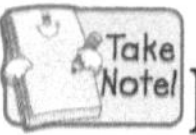

MOM DE Nutrition SO Utilize It In Health

MO – Mortality indicator
M – Morbidity indicator
D – Disability rate
E – Environmental indicator
Nutrition - Nutritional status indicator
S – Socio-economic indicator
O – Others
U – Utilization rates
It – Indicator of quality of life
In - Indicator of social and mental health
Health – Health policy indicator

8 MDG's to be achieved by 2015

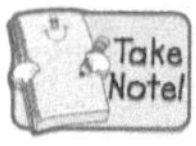

EPIDEMIC

E – Eradicate extreme poverty and hunger
P – Primary education (achieve universal primary education)
I – Improve maternal health
D– Develop a global partnership for development
E –Equality & empower women
M – Mortality (reduce child mortality)
I- I(e)nsure environmental sustainability
C – Combat HIV, malaria other

PQLI & HDI

PQLI include

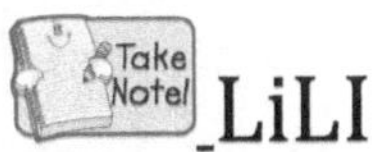 **LiLI**

Li – Life expectancy (at 1)
L - Literacy
I - IMR

HDI Include

 **LoKI**

Lo - Longevity
K – Knowledge
I - Income
EPIDEMIOLOGY

MODES OF INTERVENTION

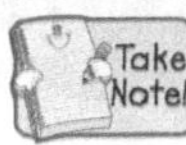 **HaS DE Yr**

Ha – Health promotion
S – Specific protection
D – Disability limitation
E – Early diagnosis and treatment
yR – Rehabilitation

TYPES OF DIRECT TRANSMISSION

 **IS DDT**

I - Inoculation
S - Soil
D – Droplet

D – Direct contact
T- Transplacental

INDIRECT TRANSMISSION

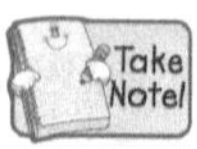 From HAVa

From – Fomite
H – Hands and finger
A – Air Born
Va – Vehicle and vector borne

GENERALLY COMMUNICABLE DISEASES ARE NOT COMMUNICABLE IN INCUBATION PERIOD EXCEPT

 CHAMPu

C - Chickenpox
HA – Hepatitis-A
M - Measles
Pu – Pertussis

CHARACTERISTIC OF CARRIER

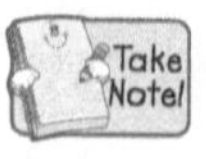 Carrier Disease ko bas [PAS] karte he

P – Presence of disease agent
A – Absence of signs and symptoms

S – Shedding of disease agent

HEALTHY CARRIERS

 SDM PoliCe

S - Salmonellosis
D- Diphtheria
M - Meningococcal meningitis
Poli - Polio
Ce – Cholera

INCUBATORY CARRIERS

 Jisne MU ME Polio drop PI HE

MU - Mumps
ME - Measles
POLIO
Drop - Diphtheria
P - Pertussis
I - Influenza
He – Hep-B

CONVALESCENT CARRIER

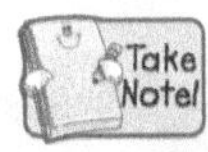 ABCD TyPe

A – Amoebic dysentery
B - Bacillary
C - Cholera
D - Diphtheria

Ty - Typhoid
Pe – Pertussis

TYPES OF RCT (Randomized Control Trial)

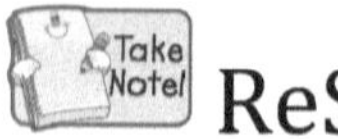 ReSPECT

Re - Risk factor trial
S – ce<u>S</u>sation trial
P – Preventive
E –Evaluation of health services
C - Clinical trial
T – Trial of etiological agent

LIVE ATTENUATED VACCINES

 Yellow TIE VaLi BMO

Yellow – Yellow fever vaccine
T - Typhoral
I - Influenza
E – Epidemic typhus
Va - Varicella
Li – Live plague
B - BCG
M – Mumps & Measles
O – OPV

USES OF EPIDEMIOLOGY

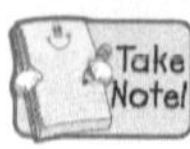 SCOPE TO Study Community S

S - Syndromic identification
Co – Completing natural history of disease
P – Planning and evaluation
E – Evaluation of individual risk and chances
To study - To study historical rise and fall of d/s
Community - Community diagnosis
S – Searching for causes and risk factor

VACCINE REACTION

BCG

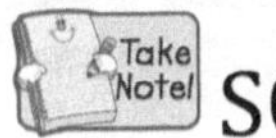 SODa

S–Suppurative lymphadenitis
O – Osteitis
Da – Disseminated Infection

Measles/MMR

FATE

F - Febrile seizures
A - Anaphylaxis
T- Thrombocytopenia
E - Encephalopathy

USES OF I.P.

 TIPS

T – Tracing the source of infection
I – Identification of point source & immunization

P – Prognosis of disease
S - Surveillance period determination

COMMUNICABLE DISEASES

USES OF STEPS IN INVESTIGATION OF AN EPIDEMIC

Verification CoDe RaDa ForTE For [44]

Verification - Verification of diagnosis
Co – Confirmation of existence of epidemic
De – Defining the population at risk
Ra – Rapid search for all cases & their characteristic
Da – Data analysis
For- Formulation of hypotheses
T– Testing of hypotheses
E – Evaluation of ecological factor
For – Further investigation

TRIAD OF CONGENITAL RUBELLA SYNDROME

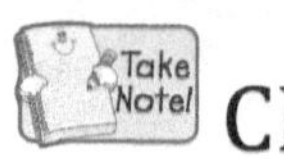

CHD

C - Cataract
H – Heart defect
D – Deafness (sensori-neural)

DIFFERENTIAL DIAGNOSIS OF AFP

 # Oral GTT

Oral – Other viruses coxsackie, ECHO, entero 70&7, mumps
G - GBS
T – Transverse myelitis
T – Traumatic neuritis

CONTROL OF STD

 ## IIMS

I – Initial planning
I - Intervention strategies
M – Monitoring and evaluation
S – Support component

4 BASIC STRATEGIES TO ERADICATE POLIO FROM INDIA

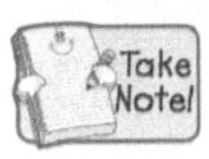 ## MAP Immunization

M – Mopping up campaign
A – AFP surveillance
P- Pulse Polio Immunization
I – Immunization (routine)

MANDATORY TESTING OF BLOOD

IS DONE FOR 5 DISEASES

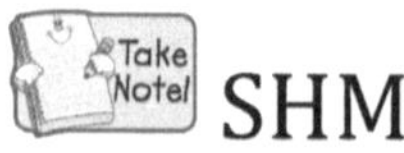 SHM

S - Syphilis
H – Hepatitis B, C & HIV
M – Malaria

DANGER SIGNS OF VERY SEVERE PNEUMONIA

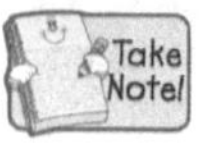 UCMS Delhi

U – Unable to drink
C - Convulsion
M – Malnutrition (severe)
S – Stridor in calm child
Delhi – Difficult to wake

HEALTH PROGRAMME

DANGER SIGNS OF CANCER

Breast ME UNEXPLAINED
EXCESSIVE BaDi SWELLING HO

BREAST – Breast lump
Me –Mole changes
UNEXPLAINED - Unexplained weight loss
EXCESSIVE – Excessive loss of blood at monthly period

Ba - Blood loss from any natural orifice
Di – Digestive change (persistent)
SWELLING – Swelling or sore that does not get better
HO – Hoarseness or cough (persistent)

MALARIA

Under MPO Annual parasite index > 2 me

 Regular TIME DE

Regular – Regular spraying
T – Treatment of cases
I – Intensify efforts in rural area
M – Malaria surveillance
E – Entomological studies
D –Decentralization of lab services
E – Establishment of DDCs & FTDs

MALARIA CONTROL STRATEGIES

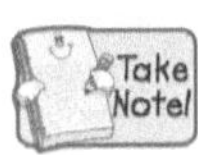 ES_2I

E - Epidemic preparedness and early response
S – Surveillance
S – Supportive intervention (CBI operational monitoring)
I – Integrated vector management (IIM)

RNTCP

SUCCESS OF DOTS DEPEND ON 5 COMPONENTS

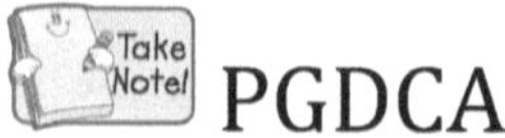 # PGDCA

P – Political commitment
G – Good quality sputum microscopy
D – Directly observed treatment
C(s) - Supply of good quality drugs (uninterrupted)
A - Accountability

SUPPORTIVE INTERVENTION

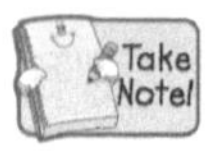 # CBI operational monitoring

C – Capacity building
B - Behavior change communication
I – Intersectoral collaboration
Operational – Operational research & field research
Monitoring – monitoring and evaluation

INTEGRATED VECTOR MANAGEMENT

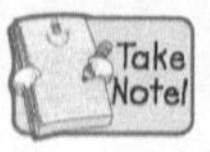 # IIM

I – Indoor residual spray
I – Insecticide treated bed nets/ LLINs
M – Measures (antilarval)

UNDER RNTCP 1ST PRIORITY IS GIVEN TO DIRECT SPUTUM EXAMINATION OF PATIENT

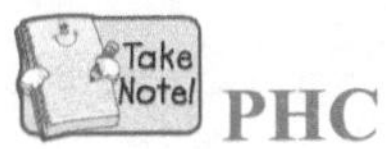 **PHC**

P – Persistent cough of about > 3 or 4wks
H - Hemoptysis
C – Continuous fever & chest pain

FALSE NEGATIVE MANTOUX TEST

 AIIMS college Pre Pg

A – Anti - allergic use
I – Immuno-suppressants use
I - hIv
M – Measles & malnutrition
College – Chicken pox
S – Severe fever
Pre - Pre-Allergic phase
Pg – Pertussis

NRHM

ROLL AND RESPONSIBILITY OF ASHA

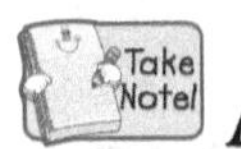 ABCDEFGHI

A– AWARENESS creation & provide information on determinants of health
B– BIRTH-PREPAREDNNESS counseling

C – Community Mobilization

D- Develop a comprehensive village health plane

E– ESCORT pregnant women/children requiring treatment & admission

F– FIRST AID and primary health care

G - Graded training to her for providing newborn care

H – Holder of essential provision for ORS, IFA, OCP, DD kit

I – Inform about birth and death

TREATMENT OF MDR T.B

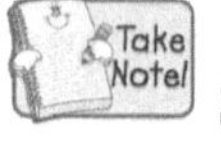 she is ok without pk - CE EZ OK for 6 months (I.P.)

C – Cycloserin

E – Ethambutol

E - Ethionamide

Z – Pyrazinamide(Z)

O - Ofloxacin

K – Kanamycin

For 18 month she is ok without pk (CE EZ OK-pk)

C - Cycloserin

E - Ethambutol

E – Ethionamide

O – Ofloxacin

GOALS OF NRHM AT COMMUNNITY LEVEL

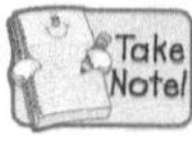 General Health Worker to Assure

Facilities and Access to Mobile Care

General – Generic drugs at subcenter & hospital level
Health – Health day at anganwadi level
Worker – Trained Worker
Assure - Assure health care at reduced financial risk
Facilities – Facilities for institutional deliveries
Access – Access to universal immunization
Mobile – Mobile Unit
Care – Good hospital care
RCH

MAIN HIGHLIGHTS OF RCH

 ICU Facility & specialist for outreach

I – INTEGRATE all intervention of fertility regulation, MCH with reproductive health
C –Client oriented & demand driven services on community need based
U – Up gradation of level of facilities for various intervention &quality care
Facility - Facility for obstetric care MTP IUD in PHC improved
Specialist - Specialist facilities for STD & RTI at all District hospital
Outreach - Outreach services for vulnerable group should improve

INTERVENTION IN SELECTED STATE

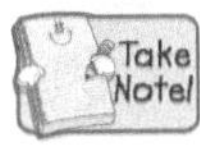 SAFE Delivery

S – SCREENING & TREATMENT OF RTI/STD
A –Additional ANM at sub centers in weak district
F – Facility or referral transport for pregnant women

E – Emergency and essential obstetric care
DELIVERY - Improve delivery services and emergency care

INTERVENTION IN ALL DISTRICT

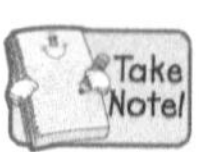 CID HE SAFE

C - CHILDHOOD SURVIVAL INTERVENTION
I - IMPLEMENTATION OF TARGET FREE APPROACH
D – DIIST. SUBPROJECT UDER LOCAL CAPACITY ENHANCEMENT
H – HIGH QUALITY TRAINING AT AAL LEVEL
E - ENHANCED COMMUNITY PARTICIPATION
S - SPECIALLY DESIGNED RCH PACKAGE
A – ADOLOSCENT HEALTH AND REPRODUCTIVE HYGIENE
F – FACILITY FOR SAFE ABORTION AT PHC
E - iEc activities

MINIMUM SERVICES BY FRU

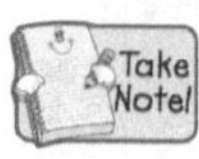 BETTER Safe Emergency Delivery of Sick newborn
B – Blood storage facility
E - Essential laboratory services
T/T – T/T of STI/RTI
R – Referral services
Safe – Safe abortion services
Emergency – Emergency obstetric care
Delivery – 24 hr delivery services
Sick - Sick children emergency care
Newborn – New-born care

IMNCI

Curative component includes Management of – DM in PSM

D - diarrhoea
M - measles
P - pneumonia
S – severe malnutrition
M – malaria

IMNCI PROCESS

 A ICTC follow-up

A - Assess
I - Identify
C - Classify
T - Treatment
C - Counsel
Follow-up - Follow-up care

HEALTH PROMOTIVE AND PREVENTIVE COMPONENT INCLUDE

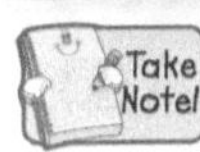 INSTa Feeding

I - Immunization
N – Nutritional counselling
S – Supplementation of iron & vit A
Ta – T/T of helminthic infestation
Feeding – Breast feeding

415NATIONAL CANCER CONTROL PROGRAMME

SCHEME UNDER REVISED PROGRAMME

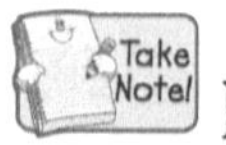 RODIE research

R – Regional cancer center scheme
O – Oncology wing development scheme
D – Decentralized NGO scheme
IEC - IEC activities at central level
Research – Research & training

NPCB

GLOBAL VISION 2020 (INCLUDE 5 DISEASES)

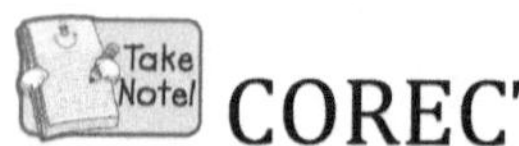 CORECT

C - Cataract
O – Onchocerciasis
Re –Refractive error
C – Childhood blindness
T - Trachoma

GOALS OF NATIONAL POPULATION POLICY

 Reduce BIPASA like girls

Reduce – 1. Infant mortality <30/1000
         2.MMR < 100/100000
B – Bring convergence in implementation of related social programme
I – INTEGRATE –
Indian system of medicine' in provision of RCH

Integration b/w management of RTI, STD & NACO
P – PROMOTE
Delayed marriage for girls
Vigorously small family norm
Prevent & control communicable d/s
A –ACHIEVE 100%
Registration of birth, death, marriage
Immunization
Delivery by trained person 80% institution
Access to information, counseling & services for fertility
Regulation & contraception
S - School education up to age 14 free & compulsory
A – Address the unmet need for basic RCH services & family planning

IDSP

SYNDROME UNDER SURVEILLANCE

JACDU fever

J - Jaundice
A - AFP
C– Cough > 3 wks
D - Diarrhea
U – Unusual event causing death/hospitalization
Fever

NATIONAL HEALTH POLICY 2002

Goals for 2005 – State IPL

State – State sector health spending increase from 5.5% to 7%
I – Integrate system of surveillance, national health accounts &

statistics
P – Polio & yaws eradication
L - Leprosy elimination

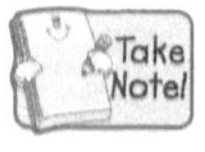 GOALS FOR 2007 - Achieve zero level of growth of HIV/AIDS

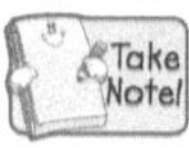 GOALS FOR 2010 –

Reduce BMI

B –blinding prevalence to 0.5%
M - Mortality by 50% due to T.B, MALRIA, VECTOR &WATER BORN disease and MMR < 100/lakh
I - IMR < 30/1000

INCREASE HEALTH UTILISATION by CENTRAL & STATE GOVT.

HEALTH – increase health expenditure %GDP from 0.9% to 2%
UTILISATION – INCREASE utilization of public health facility from < 20% to >75%
CENTRAL - INCREASE central grant to constitute of>25%
STATE - INCREASE state health spending to 8% of budget

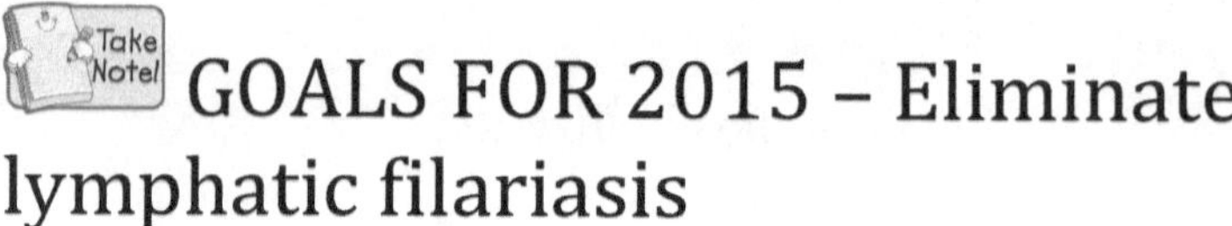 GOALS FOR 2015 – Eliminate lymphatic filariasis

OBJECTIVE OF ANTENATAL CARE

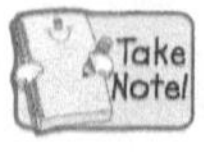 PHC remove mortality & teach

family to attend under 5

P – Promote prevent & protect maternal health
H – High risk case detection
C – Complication (to foresee complication)
Remove – Remove anxiety & dread associated with delivery
Mortality - Reduce mortality (maternal & infant)
Teach – Teach mother elements of child care
family – Family planning sensitization to mother - to attend to under 5 accompanying mothers

RISK APPROACH

HIGH RISK PREGNANACY

PPH ECLAMPSIATE wali pregnancy

P – Prolonged pregnancy (14 days after expected date)
P – Pregnancy associated with general d/s viz. CVD, kidney d/s D.M, T.B. etc
H – Hemorrhage (antepartum) & threatened abortion
E – Elderly primi (30 yrs) 7 over
C – Caesarian history
L– eLderly grand multiparas
M– Malpresentation viz. breech, transverse lie
P – Previous still-birth, intrauterine death, manual removal of placenta
S–Short statured primi (140 cm & below)
I – Instrumental & caesarian delivery history
A - Anemia
T – Twins, hydramnios
E – Eclampsia and pre-eclampsia

APGAR SCORE

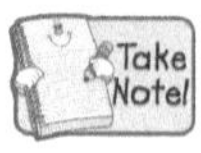 # INCLUDE BHMS reflex

B – Breathing effort
H – Heart rate
M – Muscle tone
S - Skin color
Reflex – Reflex response

DANGER SIGNALS IN PREGNANCY

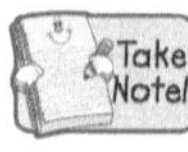 # Excessive PAIN is Not Good for Pregnancy

Excessive - Excessive BLEEDING OR SHOW DURING LABOUR
P – Post-partum hemorrhage or collapse during labour
A – A TEMPERATURE OF 38 C OR OVER during labour
I – Irregular slow or excessively fast foetal rate
N –No or sluggish pain after membrane rupture
Is Not - Not separated placenta within ½ hour
Good - Good pain but no progress after membrane rupture
For Pregnancy – Prolapse of cord or hand

MCH INDICATOR

 # PSM Family

P – Prevalence of low birth weight babies
S – services (immunization, ANC, delivery)
M - mortality indicator
(MMR, perinatal, neonatal, infant, under 5)
Family – family planning indicator (crude birth rate, TFR, CPR)

MEDICAL CAUSES OF MATERNAL MORTALITY

 **India TO Unsafe HE for AAM aadmi**

OBSTETRIC causes

India - Infection
TO – Toxemias of pregnancy
Unsafe – Unsafe abortion
HE - Hemorrhage

NON-OBSTRETIC causes

A - Anemia
A - Accidents
M - Malignancy
Aadmi – Associated diseases

USES OF GROWTH CHART

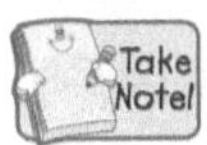 **GDP Evaluation Tool**

G – Growth monitoring
D – Diagnostic tool
P – Planning & policy making
Evaluation Tool– Tool for teaching, education& action

Preventive and social measure to reduce MMR

Early ANC Dau For PREVENTION/ Treatment of malaria & Clean Safe

Delivery

Early – Early registration of pregnancy
ANC - ANC checkup at least 3
Dau – Dietary supplement
For – Family planning promotion
Prevention - Prevention of complication
Treatment – Treatment of medical condition
Malaria – Malaria & tetanus prophylaxis
Clean – Clean delivery practices
Safe – Safe abortion
Delivery – Institutional delivery for women with bad obstetric history delivery by trained dais & FHW

FACTOR AFFECTING INFANT MORTALITY

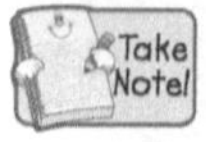 BIOLOGICAL – BAM He

B –Birth weight, order, space
A – Age of mother
M – Multiple birth
He – High fertility & family size

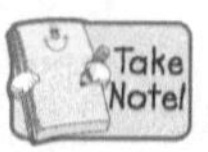 CULTURAL & SOCIAL FACTOR – B3REAST

B – Breast feeding
B – Brutal habits
B – Broken families
R - Religion
E – Early marriages & education of mother
A - A(e)nviornmental sanitation
S – Sex of child
T – quali**T**y mothering and health care

PREVENTION OF PERINATAL & INFANT

NUTRITION

 ## SAFE Nutritious Feeding

S – Sanitation
A – Access to PHC
F – Family planning
E – Education
Nutritious – Prenatal nutrition
Feeding - Breast feeding

ICDS SERVICES

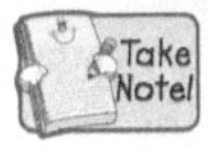 ## SHINER

S – Supplementary nutrition
H - Health checkup
I - Immunization
N – Nutrition &health education
E –Education (nonformal)
R - Referral services

EPIDEMIOLOGICAL ASSESSMENT OF IODINE DEFICIENCY

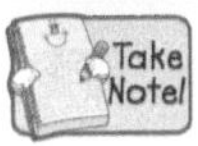 ## Measurement of neonatal ECG

Measurement – Measurement of TSH & T4
Neonatal – Neonatal hypothyroidism

E – EXCRETION OF IODINE IN URINE
C – Cretinism prevalence
G – Goiter prevalence

CONDITIONALLY ESSENTIAL AMINO ACID

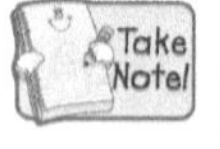 CyTy GATE

Cy - CYSTEINE
Ty - TYROSINE
G – Glutamine & glycine
A - Arginine
T – Taurine

TESTS OF PASTEURIZED MILK

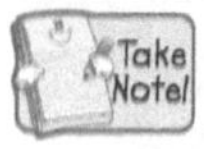 PSC

P – Phosphatase test
S – Standard plate count
C – Coliform count

ENVIORNMENT

TYPES OF SANITORY LATRINE (NON-SERVICE

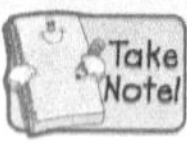 Water-seal SABD

Water-seal - Water-seal type
S – Septic tank
A - Aqua privy

B – Bore hole
D – Dug well

METHODS OF TEMPORARY HARDNESS

 **BAAP**

B - Boiling
A – Addition of lime
A – Addition of sodium carbonate
P – Permutit process

AIR HUMIDITY IS MEASURED BY

 **SAHyD**

S – Sling/whirling psychrometer
A – Assman psychrometer
Hy – Hygrometer
D – Dry & wet bulb thermometer

CHEMICAL INDICATOR OF AIR POLLUTION

 **GASCoefficient**

G – Grit & dust measurement
A – Air pollution index
S – Sulphur dioxide & soiling index
C – Coefficient of haze

AUTOSOMAL DOMINANT TRAITS

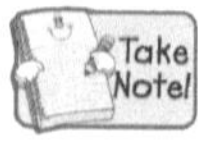

NRHM He AK politics

N - NEUROFIBROMATOSIS
R –RETINOBALASTOMA
H - HUNTINGTONS CHOREA
M – MARFANS SYNDROME
HE – HEREDITARY SPHEROCYTOSIS &
HYPERLIPOPROTEINEMIA I, II, III, IV
AK – ACHONNDROPLASIA
POLYTICS – POLYPOSIS COLI & POLYCYSTIC KIDNEY

PREVENTION OF OCCUPATIONL DISEASES

MEDICAL MEASURES

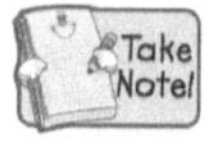

Pyar ME NO SUPERVISION Pyar needs Maintenance & Counseling

PyaR – Pre-placental examination
ME – Medical and health care services
NO - Notification
SUPERVISION - Supervision of working environment
Pyar – Periodic examination
Needs Maintenance – Maintenance and analysis of record
Counseling – Counseling and health education

ENGINEERING MEASURES

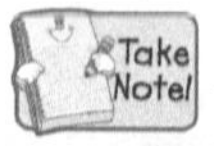

DESI GIRL ME PEM

D – Design of building & dust control
E – Environmental monitoring
S - Substitution
I - Isolation
GI - Good housekeeping & ventilation
R - Research
L – Local exhaust ventilation
Me - Mechanization
P – Protective devices
E - Enclosure
M – Monitoring of statistics

CATAGORIES OF BIOMEDICAL WASTE

 HAM Se DES SOLID he

H – Human anatomical waste
A – Animal waste
M – Microbiological & bio-technology waste
Se – Sharp waste
De – Discarded medicine
S – Solid waste
So – Soiled waste
L - Liquid ash
ID – Incineration ash
HE – cHEmical waste

BENEFITS TO EMPLOYESS UNDERR ESI

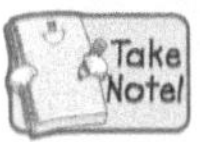 Sickness Me Money REFUND Deta he ESI

Sickness – Sickness benefit

Me – Medical benefit
Money - Maternity benefit
Re – Rehabilitation allowance
Fun – Funeral expenses
D – Disability benefit
Deta he – Dependents benefit

MANAGEMENT METHOD BASED ON BEHAVIORAL SCIENCE

 OPIUM

O – Organizational design
P - Personal management
I – Information system
U - commUnication
M – MBO

SOCIO-ECONOMI SCALE

URBAN

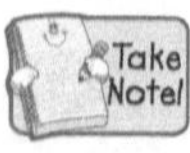 MuKeSh Ji

Mu- Modified kuppu
Ke - Kulshreshtha
Sh - Srivastava
Ji – Jalota

RURAL

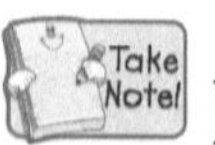 RaMU Sir

Ra- Radhukar
M- Modified B.G. Prasad
U – Udai pareek
S – Shirpurkar

HEALTH PLANNING AND MANAGEMENT ELEMENTS OF PHC

 **ELEMENTS**

E – Education concerning health problem & their control
L – Locally endemic d/s prevention &control
E – Essential drugs
M – MCH care including family planning
E – EPI (immunization) against disease
N – Nutrition & proper food supply promotion
T – T/T of common d/s and injuries
S – Safe water supply& sanitation

IOB OF MEDICAL OFFICER AT PHC

 **VICO**

V – Visit
School in PHC area
Subcenters
I – Implement
UIP
IMNCI
C – Captain of health team
O – Organize
Training of health personnel
Staff meeting
Vasectomy & tubectomy camp

FUNCTION OF PHC

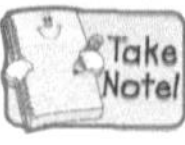 **Safe ManageMent(M/M) By RNTCP**

Safe – Safe water supply & basic sanitation
M –Medical care
M – MCH including family planning
By - Basic laboratory services
R – Referral services
N – National health programme
T – Training
C - Collection and reporting of vital statistics
P – Prevention and control of locally endemic disease

STAFFING PATTERN AT PHC

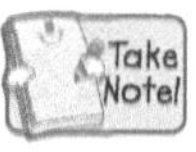 **PHC Lab 2 HEAD 1 Medical Officer 3 ki wife 5 class (iv) HA(he)**

PHC lab – **P**harmacist, **H**ealth assistant, **C**lerk, **Lab** technician – **2**
HEAD –**H**ealth worker, **E**ducator, **A**ccount manager, **D**river-1
MO-3
Mid-wiFe– **f**ive Class 4 – 4 HA - AYUSH - 1 TOTAL – **25/24**

SRIVASTAV COMMITTEE

Srivastav committee DRIVER create kiye HE

D – Development of 'referral services complex'
R - ROME
I – Infrastructure (3 tier rural health)

V – Village health guide
ER – Establishment of medical & health education commission
Create – Create 'bands of para-professional & semi-professional health worker
He – Health worker (MHW, HA)

WORK OF W.H.O

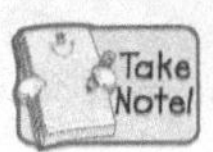

PDF HE BHaI

P – Prevention & control of specific d/s
D – Development of comprehensive health services
F – Family health
H – Health statistics
E – Environmental health
B – Bio-medical research
HaI – Health literature and Information

VOLUNTARY HEALTH AGENCIES IN INDIA

BHARTI Central Kasturba family board B – bharat sevak samaj

H – Hind Kusht Nivaran Sangh
A – All India women's conference
R – Red cross (Indian)
T – Tuberculosis association India
I – Indian council for child welfare
Central – Central social welfare board
Kasturba –Kasturba memorial fund
Family – Family planning association India
Board – Blind relief society & bodies (professional)

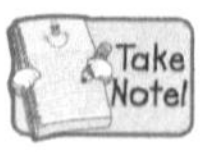 # 1000 population par VAT lagta he

V – Village health guide
A - ASHA
T – Trained Dai/TBA

LIST OF QURANTINABLE DISEASES

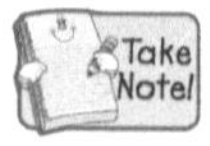 # Ye VIP D/S he

Ye – Yellow fever
V – Viral hemorrhagic fever
I – Infectious T.B.
P - Plague
D - Diphtheria
S – Smallpox & SARS

DISEASES UNDER INTERNATIONAL HEALTH

REGULATUON (IHR)

 # WHY So Serious CoP

W – Wild polio
H – Human influenza
Y – Yellow fever
So – Small pox Serious - SARS
Co - Cholera
P – Plague

DISEASES UNDER INTERNATIONAL SURVEILANCE

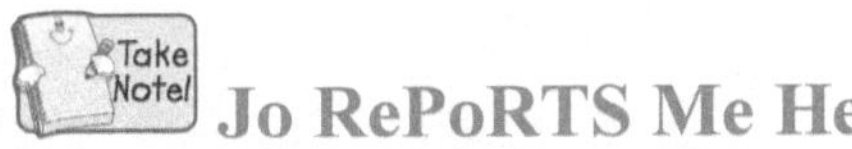

Jo RePoRTS Me He

Re – Relapsing fever
Po - Polio
R - Rabies
T – Typhus fever (louse born)
S - Salmonellosis
Me - Malaria
He – Human influenza

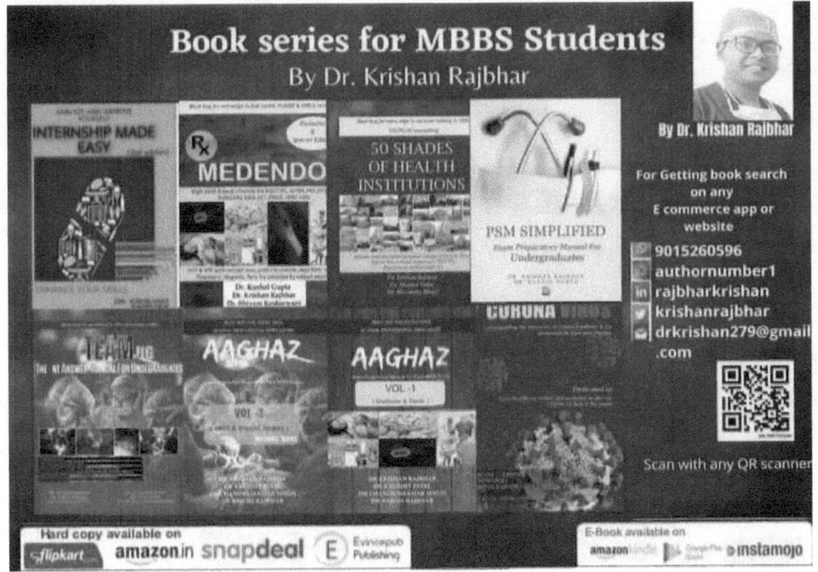

9 789354 463174